Stop Your Day

Top 10 Health Conditions
Busy Women Need to Stop
Ignoring and Start Preventing

By: Dr. Beth Westie
&
Deja Dircks

Stop Your Day

Dr. Beth Westie
4024 Blackhawk Rd
Eagan, MN 55122
www.stopyourday.com
Ordering Information:
Quantity sales. Special discounts are available on quantity purchases by corporations, associations, and others. For details, contact the publisher at the address above.
Orders by U.S. trade bookstores and wholesalers. Please contact Dr. Beth Westie: Tel: (651) 402-5910 or email info@stopyourday.com.

Printed in the United States of America

Disclaimer Page

This book is not intended as a substitute for the medical advice of physicians. The reader should regularly consult a physician in matters relating to his/her health, and particularly with respect to any symptoms that may require diagnosis or medical attention.

Stop Your Day

Table of Contents

Health Conditions:

About the Authors

Dr. Beth Westie was born and raised on a small goat farm in Eagan, Minnesota. After being on the Eagan Wildcat team that collected two state volleyball titles, her sights turned to higher education. Being the recipient of a full athletic and academic scholarship to Northern Michigan University, she was able to combine her passion for women's health along with her love of sport, playing volleyball for the NMU Wildcats. Upon graduating NMU with a bachelor's in biology and physiology, the blossoming massage therapist promptly enrolled in the chiropractic program at Minnesota's Northwestern Health Sciences University. Only after becoming a mother of two (now three), as well as a certified acupuncturist and a Doctor of Chiropractic, Beth could finally focus on a career path. This is when her passion for women's health and wellness rose, and she could work to educate and transform the lives of women around the world.

Deja Dircks was born in Shakopee, Minnesota. A childhood filled with various activities and athletics lead the way to her Bachelor's degree in Exercise Science with a minor in sports medicine at the University of Minnesota at Mankato. Here is where Deja began her love for running. She has completed several major marathons, including notables such as the New York City Marathon; with her sights set on the Chicago Marathon later this fall, and the London Marathon next spring. After graduation, Deja pursued her interest in the health and wellness field, beginning work at a chiropractic clinic. After spending nearly five years assisting in patient care in the clinic, she has teamed her passions with Dr. Westie to focus on the health and wellness of women. Together, Deja and Dr. Westie are creating new ideas and awareness when it comes to health and wellness in women.

Introduction

No woman has ever said, "I have three kids that are in lots of activities, a career where I manage others, and a household to run. I could really use a few more things on my plate."

People are busy, especially women. We pack as much into our day as possible, and then try to squeeze in a little bit more. We rush from one activity to the next, barely taking a minute to catch our breath. Anytime a family member or friend has a crisis, we know exactly how to jump in and help, doing so while rearranging our own schedule to make it all work by the end of the day.

I have seen women scrap their entire plan for the day at a moment's notice, and rush to the aid of others. As a busy mom of three young kids, it seems almost daily I do it myself. It sometimes starts within the first minutes of the day. I wake up at five with the determination of getting to the gym and back before my husband has to leave for work, and the kids wake up. That leaves me with about thirty minutes of "quiet" time to get ready—but suddenly I hear a screech from upstairs. My youngest has a bloody nose, leaving a mess everywhere. Immediately I jump into the caretaker role. First I stop the bleeding, start the bath, and then washer for the soiled sheets. Once my little one is dry, and in clean jammies, I can tuck her back in a clean bed for an hour or so. There went my gym time.

"Oh well," I say to myself,' "there's always tomorrow." I envision that I will be able to sneak away to the gym tonight, but secretly know that's wishful thinking. I have a full schedule the rest of the day, and I may get too tired and forget my goal.

Health Plans and Self-care

In this hectic life, it's almost too easy to get off course with your health plans and self-care, and keeping on task has been shown to be the most important factor in attaining and maintaining your health in every area. Putting yourself and your health first is a great mindset to have, and extremely important, but often it feels like a very unrealistic motto for busy women to live by. Often women put up with a health issue of some kind for too long because they have too much on their plate. It can be tough to remember to take your daily vitamins when you are trying to get kids ready in the morning, and it never fails—one misses the bus, while the other one who made the bus forgot her lunch.

I have treated women that have put up with horrible headaches for five or more years because they have to work, and then rush kids to soccer practice. Only when the headache gets so bad that it causes blurred vision and driving becomes near impossible, does she make herself a priority, and actually seek help. The problem has been going on for such a long time, it has now become more difficult to treat. The only time these busy women will give in and seek professional help is when it stops them from doing the normal day-to-day things.

About This Book Geared Towards Women...

Some of the information in this book may seem intense. Some of the facts might startle you, but the goal is to get you thinking about your own health. I haven't written this just to present facts or sugarcoat anything. I am very passionate about educating women on how healthy choices can greatly impact their lives. I believe with this information you will be able to take swift action with your health—and the health of other important women in your lives. In all honesty, it could save your life.

You will see a trend in both preventing and also caring for all these dangerous conditions for women. I want to address this at the beginning because as you read it over and over in the following pages, I don't want it to get diluted. The truth is the regular daily activities that are focused on better health and have the biggest impact are:

- Exercise. Get your body moving, using any form of activity you enjoy, and try new things. At least 30 minutes a day, 4-5 days a week is necessary.
- Eat healthy food. Eat a diet of whole foods that are as fresh as possible and limit the amount of processed foods. If you can't grow it or kill it, try to cut it out.
- Eat more vegetables. If you don't like veggies, find them in a powder or supplement. Is it as good as the fresh? No, but it's better than not eating them.
- Say "NO" more often; to extra tasks or errands that you don't need to add to your to do list.
- Take the time to care for yourself. If you feel like you need more information, reach out for more resources. Read books, watch videos on-line, and talk with others who have great health. Just get started...and do it today.

It is my mission for this book to reach women worldwide so they can awaken themselves to the biggest dangers affecting their health. It starts with education on the top 10 conditions for women and when you *need* to put yourself first.

Don't miss these signs and symptoms that can save your time, money, and your life because you were too busy to pay attention.

Health Condition No. 1:
Heart Disease

I had a heart attack, and didn't even know it!

I am a 40-year-old mother of two. Besides being busy with my family, I own a small hair salon. For the past couple of years I have made an extra effort to eat a cleaner diet, always buying organic fruits and vegetables when possible. I joined a community workout group and we exercise five days a week. Over the past couple years, my salon has become quite popular, requiring more of my time and attention. But like they say, "Being busy is good!" Along with my growing family, and successful business I have also been caring for my aging parents, leaving little time for me to focus solely on myself. Let's be honest, do any busy working mothers have time just to themselves?

After a morning hike with a couple of my friends, I was feeling exhausted and more fatigued than normal. As any busy woman would, I carried on with my daily routine of getting the kids to school, heading to the salon to check in on everything, stopping at the grocery store, making sure I had snacks ready for when I pick the kids up from school, which was right before dropping them off at soccer practice. Throughout the day I started to notice some nausea and dizziness, but I honestly thought it might be because I hadn't eaten a lot that day.

After spending the day feeling like I was moving at a thousand miles per hour, I noticed the nausea had increased while lying in bed. The next morning I decided to skip my work out because I was still feeling dizzy, and even more nauseous. After realizing my symptoms had continued to get worse for a third day, I decided it was time to head into the doctor to get it checked out because it was keeping me from carrying on with my normal routine. After having multiple tests, my doctor came into the room to give me the scariest news I've ever gotten. I had a heart attack three days ago, and now as a result of waiting to get to the doctor, it has caused some permanent heart damage, which puts me at risk for having additional heart attacks in the future. All because I was too busy to get my symptoms checked out.

● Every 90 seconds a woman suffers a heart attack in the United States, making heart disease the No. 1 killer of women.

● 1 in 3 women die from heart disease, and the most common cause is a narrowing or blockage of an artery.

What is Heart Disease?

Heart disease covers a range of conditions that affect your heart, including coronary artery disease, heart arrhythmias, and heart defects. Cardiovascular disease, which includes narrowed or blocked arteries, is the most common form of heart disease.

What Should I Look For?

Often, the first symptom of a heart attack *is death*. The signs and symptoms of heart disease frequently present themselves very differently in men than in women. Now read that again. Most people are familiar with the classic male symptoms:

- chest pain
- shortness of breath
- pain in the left arm.

Women may have the same symptoms, but more often heart disease presents with:

- nausea or vomiting

- back pain
- jaw pain
- fatigue
- dizziness or lightheadedness
- indigestion or heartburn.

The tricky part is how to know the difference between signs of something serious and a simple illness, because we all feel sick at some point. When experiencing nausea or fatigue, someone with any number of those risk factors is going to say, "Well! That's me every other day," or "Golly, That's normal for me." This is why it is so difficult to diagnose heart disease in women. It also makes it even more important to know exactly what signs to look for, and when to stop your day, and take the next step to getting help.

Other Conditions to Rule Out:

Heart disease can be tough to recognize when some of the symptoms and signs previously listed above are vague. It's easy to point the finger of blame on something else that is less serious—but this is where the danger lies for women. Often women will experience symptoms of vomiting, fatigue, and some back pain, and *not knowing they are in danger*—think, "I must have caught a bug. I

should just lie down, and I'll feel better soon, but I have to get to my kid's baseball game tonight."
Symptoms of heart disease that can be misidentified are: musculoskeletal pain (body pain), flu, and other illness.

What Puts Me More at Risk?

Consider these top risk factors when experiencing the symptoms listed above:

- Diabetes
- Diet that is high in saturated fat* and cholesterol
- Excessive alcohol consumption
- High cholesterol
- High blood pressure
- Obesity
- Physical inactivity
- Tobacco use
- Family history of heart disease.

* Saturated fat is found in animal products like fatty meats, lard, butter, cheese, whole milk, cream, and oils.

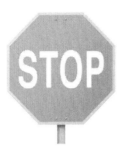

Stop Your Day

When you experience one or more of these signs and symptoms and you aren't feeling better after a day. *Do not delay, see your doctor and get checked.*

Diagnostic Tests:

These numbers may not sound very exciting, but they are extremely important. Knowing these benchmarks can greatly decrease your risk of heart disease.

- Blood Pressure – normal is 120/80.
- Cholesterol – total cholesterol is normal below 200mg/dL
- LDL (Bad Cholesterol) is normal below 130mg/dL
- HDL(Good Cholesterol) is normal above 60mg/dL
- Triglycerides are normal below 150mg/dL and even better if it's below 100mg/dL.

How Do I Prevent Heart Disease—and Other Health Concerns?

Most forms of heart disease can be prevented and/or treated with healthy lifestyle choices.

- Regular exercise is vital at least 4-5 days a week for at least 30 minutes. High Intensity Interval Training (H.I.I.T.) is a great way to get a workout in a short amount of time, and my favorite way to do that is with tabatas. Tabatas are circuit exercises you perform for about 20 seconds followed by a 10 second break and then repeat. You can do them anywhere, with little or no equipment (check out multiple resources online, or check the back of the book for more ideas). Pilates, yoga, jogging, dancing, weight lifting, or any movement is beneficial for your heart and disease prevention...just get moving.
- Nutrition is almost more important than exercise. You can't out-exercise a bad diet. Getting healthy fats daily, like omegas from fish oils, ensures you're getting the healthy fats your body needs.

Be sure to eat 5 servings of veggies a day, especially leafy greens. This may seem like a lot, but you will quickly notice a big improvement in your health.

- Your oral health, including your gums, can have a huge impact on your heart health. Make sure to get regular dental care and floss daily.

It really is that simple to protect your heart.

Here are some other things to do:

1. Getting a massage on a regular basis, as often as once a week to once a month, also prevents heart disease. It can increase blood flow and decrease blood pressure, which can have an immediate positive impact on your heart health. If you've never had a massage, or had regular massage, now is the time to try it.

2. Take your vitamins. It can be tough in a busy world to get all the nutrients your body needs from just the food you eat, so a vitamin is a great insurance policy. The top four supplements to take daily are:

3. Multivitamin – that is made from organic whole food sources, and from a company that has tested the supplements by an independent third party. This assures the vitamin is of a high quality and has the best absorption rate and bioavailability.

4. Fish Oil – from a pure source. You usually get what you pay for on this one, so make sure the source is clean and not contaminated, or you do not receive any benefit from the fish oil.

5. Probiotic – one that needs to be refrigerated ensures that the bacteria are the most alive, which sounds weird, but is actually good. Probiotics have live cultures which help to break down your food and make digestion easier.

6. Vitamin D – most people in the U.S. are deficient in Vitamin D, so get your levels checked, and make sure you are taking enough.

Most people find they will need to increase their daily intake. Recent studies have shown that people benefit from taking large doses (2,000-5,000 IU/day)

Heart Disease prevention is an important daily activity, and the more you do to take care of yourself, the less it will Stop Your Day!

NOTE: All the above points are great recommendations to improve all aspects of your health, not just heart disease (this will be reinforced in other sections).

Questions to Ask Yourself:

Does anyone in your immediate family have heart disease?

Has your doctor commented about your heart being a concern?

Are you already using medications for heart disease?

Have you changed anything in your life related to concerns about your heart?

Were you aware women's symptoms were different than men's?

Do you know your blood pressure readings?

Do you know what your cholesterol levels are?

When is the last time you had a physical?

Have you ever experienced heart-related symptoms that you've "ignored"?

Stop Your Day

Health Condition No. 2:
Lung Cancer

I had lung cancer for months before I finally paid attention.

I had built a life many women would dream of--a loving husband, three amazing kids, and a successful job that allowed me to work from home most days. Although I love this busy lifestyle, sometimes I feel like I thrive off the stress. In early January, I decided we were going to escape the cold and take the kids to a warmer climate for a week or so. I immediately jumped into planning mode. I had booked the flights, hotel room, notified the school, and found some exciting things to do while we were there. Of course I did all this planning while working, packing lunches for kids, making sure homework was done, feeding the dogs, and kissing my husband good-bye for the day. Doesn't every women work this way?

Two days before we were leaving, during a rare minute to myself, I realized I had a nagging cough. It was nothing too bad, so I decided to down some Vitamin C, and carry on with my day, because honestly, that's all the time I had.

Three months later my husband says, "Jeez, you still have that cough from winter. Maybe you should get it checked out." until that point, 1 almost hadn't even noticed that it was still hanging around. 1 have always been healthy and never smoked. 1 took his advice and went to the doctor. Besides the cough, which really didn't bother me, as it was more annoying than anything else, 1 felt normal. 1 was slightly more fatigued, but figured, who isn't when they are juggling a family, work, and life? 1 was given antibiotics and sent on my way. 1 was confident 1 would finally kick the cough.

Another four months later, and 1 realized the cough is still lingering, and I'm starting to feel even more fatigued than before. Maybe this was because 1 had recently been promoted, now working longer hours, and was more stressed with trying to manage a larger team of people. My husband, who again was the voice of reason, mentioned that 1 should probably see my doctor again.

When the doctor came into the room 1 could tell something was wrong, but what could this stupid cough have possibly lead to? This time my doctor's words were life changing, and when she said "lung cancer", 1 looked around to make sure she was talking to me. Yep, she was. 1 was so confused. How could this happen? 1 felt like 1 was overall fairly young and healthy. Not only did I have lung cancer, but it was already stage 4, and had spread throughout my whole body. I am now facing some major treatments—and the real possibility of leaving my kids without a mom—all because I didn't take the time to notice a lingering cough.

- Lung cancer is the #1 cancer killer of women and causes more deaths than breast cancer, uterine cancer, and ovarian cancer combined.
- 1 in 5 women who get diagnosed with lung cancer have never touched a cigarette.
- Lung cancer is the most common cancer worldwide, and almost 160,000 Americans are expected to die in 2015. (Lung cancer related deaths per year for women continues to rise while that rate has plateaued for men)
- 57% of cases are diagnosed at stage 4.

What is Lung Cancer?

Lung cancer is a cancer that forms in the tissues of the lungs. *Squamous cell lung cancer* is more common in men, and *adenocarcinoma* is more common in women. Lung cancer can move through the body very quickly. The five-year survival rate is 54% when the cancer is diagnosed in the early stages, which only happens in about *1 out of every 7 people diagnosed*, which are terrible odds.

What Are the Symptoms?

This is another disease that can be really tough to identify for women. With cancer, most people think of a lump they find on their body. Lung cancer can present with just a persistent cough and not many other symptoms; leading people to put off making an appointment because the cough doesn't appear to be too serious. Other things to pay attention to are:

- fatigue
- malaise (feeling ill)
- body aches
- gradual shortness of breath
- back pain or neck pain

These symptoms can be slightly vague, and seem like they are not a big deal, so the biggest one to pay attention to is the cough that won't go away after 3 to 4 weeks.

Other Conditions to Rule Out:

It's easy to mistake some of the symptoms for a simple cold or flu. Other illnesses to rule out would be bronchitis or pneumonia, that cause fluid in the lungs, some type of infection, allergies or something else very mild.

What Puts Me More at Risk?

The greatest risk factor for lung cancer is smoking. The longer you have smoked in relation to the number of cigarettes smoked per day greatly increases your odds of being diagnosed. Other exposures such as radon or industrial fumes can also heighten the risk. But the most important one is smoking. Don't start, and if you have, stop.

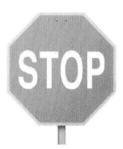

Stop Your Day

If you do smoke or have ever smoked, and have a cough that won't go away after 3–4 weeks, you might have some worrisome thoughts about lung cancer when making an appointment to see your doctor. It's the person who has never smoked,

29

who thinks they couldn't possibly have lung cancer that waits the longest. The more time that has passed before a diagnosis, the more difficult lung cancer is to treat. If you have had a cough for more than 3–4 weeks, regardless of smoking history, see your doctor. Make the time to get checked. Remember, only 15% of people get diagnosed in the early stage of the disease. If you wait, your chances of survival *go down greatly.*

Diagnostic Tests:

It's really helpful if you know your family's health history, and whether lung cancer is present, but ultimately your own health history and smoking history is of the most value. Know your body, and if you do have a cough that won't go away, please don't dismiss it.

A CT scan or x-ray can pick up lesions in the lungs, but it is a sample of tissue – either from sputum or a biopsy – examined under a microscope that confirms the diagnosis.

How Do I Prevent Lung Cancer?

- The best way to prevent lung cancer is to not smoke. So, don't smoke.
- Your overall health also plays a part. Here comes the healthy diet and exercise

part again. To prevent lung cancer and boost your overall health, nutrition is going to be key. Focus on lots of leafy greens. If you don't like leafy greens and aren't a fan of salads, find a way to get them into your system. Figure out what works for you. There are ways to juice or mix them with other vegetables, or in a protein shake where you can't taste them as much. As an alternative, get powdered greens you can mix with water or other beverages and get them into your body.

- Exercise should be focused on the High Intensity Interval Training (H.I.I.T.) as well. It's the fastest way to increase your lung capacity, and get in a great workout. Try alternating H.I.I.T. with a 20-minute walk every other day.
- Take your vitamins daily – see examples in Heart Disease section.

**All these recommendations are helpful for preventing all types of cancer.
The healthier you are, the better chance you have if you do get diagnosed.**

Questions to Ask Yourself:

Has anyone in your family been diagnosed with lung cancer?

Have you been experiencing a cough that hasn't gone away in three or more weeks?

Do you smoke or have you smoked?

Have you been around smoke or other chemical fumes?

When was your last physical?

Health Condition No. 3: Diabetes

I ignored my diagnosis because I was sure I was going to be fine.

My first pregnancy was so easy; almost too easy, and I was ecstatic when I found out I was pregnant with my second child. We knew we wanted to expand our family, but first I wanted to lose a little more weight before having another baby. I was going to focus on that in the next few months, but we were pleasantly surprised a little early. Then again, doesn't it always happen that way? Even though I always heard that no two pregnancies are ever the same, I was sure that didn't apply to me. This one started out exactly like the first one did, no morning sickness, no serious cravings, and even more energy than normal. I know, some of you reading this probably hate me a little right now, but that's honestly how it was for me. It was almost a treat to be pregnant.

At my six-month checkup, I was tested for gestational diabetes. Honestly I didn't think anything of it, because it was the same standard test as with my first child. I weighed more with this pregnancy, but I was sure it was because I was heavier at the time I conceived. When the doctor told me the test was positive for gestational diabetes, I was shocked. Everything else was pretty much the same, how could this be so different? Initially I thought maybe there was a mistake with the test. I didn't take it seriously at all. I had fully sunk into enjoying pregnancy, and thought I would just worry about the weight issue after the baby was born.

Little did I know then that the next ten weeks of ignoring the diagnosis would drastically change not only my life, but also the life of my baby. My baby was born premature with respiratory distress syndrome, and I now I have type 2 diabetes.

- 29 million Americans have diabetes.
- Women with diabetes are more likely to have a heart attack, and at a younger age. In adults over the age of 20, more than 1 in every 10 people have diabetes
- More than a third of those aged 20 and over are pre-diabetic.
- Diabetes is on the rise at a dangerous pace. In 2010, 26 million Americans were diabetic, which has climbed to over 29

million in 2014 — a huge increase in just four years.

- 1 in 4 people don't realize they have the disease, which makes it all the more dangerous as it severely increases the risk of heart disease, stroke, blindness, kidney failure, and amputation of toes.

What is Diabetes?

Diabetes is the body's inability to control the amount of sugar in the bloodstream because the body doesn't produce enough or doesn't properly use insulin. The two types of diabetes: Type 1 and Type 2.

- Type 1 is an autoimmune disease where the pancreas stops producing insulin on its own. About 5% to 10% of people are diagnosed with Type 1.
- Type 2 is insulin resistant. This occurs when the body makes too much insulin in response to having too much sugar in the bloodstream. Over a period of time too much sugar is consumed for the body to process, but the pancreas can't keep up with that pace, so the cells burn out then fail, and then can't produce enough insulin to lower the sugar levels in the

35

bloodstream. It takes years to develop into full blown type 2 diabetes.

What Should I Look For?

Some of the most common signs are:

- frequent urination
- increased thirst and hunger
- tiredness
- lack of interest in activities
- difficulty concentrating
- tingling sensation or numbness in hands or feet
- blurred vision
- slow-healing cuts

With this list of symptoms, you may not think you are diabetic simply because if you are tired, have slow-healing cuts, and increased thirst, it probably won't seem like they are linked symptoms, and you can miss these cues indicating you may have a serious problem.

Other Conditions to Rule Out:

With some diabetic symptoms people often think they have a cold or flu, which has made them tired. Most of the time, when people fail to get diagnosed and treated for diabetes, they think their symptoms are mild and not related to the disease.

What Puts Me More at Risk?

Your weight and diet are the biggest risk factors for Type 2. Diabetes does not show up overnight. You're not going to wake up tomorrow with Type 2 diabetes because you ate ice cream today. It's a slow process that takes time to show itself. Poor daily nutrition and poor exercise habits are the biggest risk factors.

Family history is also a reason to be concerned about Type 1. High blood pressure and elevated triglycerides also add to the risk of diabetes.

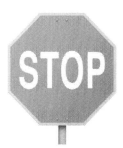

Stop Your Day

Experiencing increased thirst, frequent urination, increased hunger and fatigue are reasons to get in to your doctor immediately.

Diagnostic Tests:

Blood sugar numbers are important to track. Fasting glucose level tells you your blood sugar level when you haven't eaten for at least 8 hours. A normal fasting glucose is 100mg/dL or less. Getting this blood test at least every three years, can change your life. Tracking your weight and body-fat percentage can help to maintain healthy blood sugar levels.

How Do I Prevent Diabetes?

You can do nothing to prevent Type 1 Diabetes, but you can manage it. Type 1 diabetes is best managed by:

- Keeping BMI within the normal range of 18.5-14.9.
- Non-inflammatory diet that eliminates gluten, dairy, sugar and red meat
- Regular exercise 4-5 days a week for 30 minutes.

Data has shown that type 2 diabetes is preventable in 9 out of 10 cases by maintaining a normal BMI, exercising for 30 minutes 4-5 days a week and a healthy diet.

Type 2 diabetes is manageable once it has onset by the same as above recommendations.

Many health improvements can be made with losing just 5%–7% of your body weight if you are overweight or obese. Being active for as little as 22 minutes a day can improve outcomes for this disease.

Nutrition for diabetes is very important because it allows you to prevent and help treat the disease.

Questions to Ask Yourself:

Does anyone in your family have diabetes? What type?

Has your doctor commented about your blood sugar being too high, or recommended dietary changes?

Have you changed anything in your life related to concerns about your blood sugar?

Do you know what your "fasting" blood sugar number is?

When was your last physical?

Health Condition No. 4:

Stress

My stress caused my life to spiral out of control before I even realized it.

My family used to call me their rock, mostly because I was always able to handle a lot of stress without showing it or feeling like it really affected me. It seemed like no matter what happened, I could always find the solution to any problem, and fix it before it caused too much unnecessary stress. I carried this mantra with me into my first job, which ultimately made me a great success. I moved up the corporate ladder quickly. In my mid-20s, I was already a well-respected executive, in a multi-million dollar company. Getting in the groove of managing a team of people, while also raising two kids and trying to keep the house standing, took a little more time than I had expected, but eventually I felt like everything was under control.

I can distinctly remember the day we had our monthly executive meeting, and the CEO of the company stood at the front of the room and told us we were going to be downsizing. Over half my team was going to be eliminated, and I was going to be taking on most of the responsibility of not only laying off these people, but also picking up their workload. In terms of stress, this was bigger than anything I had ever experienced before. I knew this was something I could handle and I was determined to achieve my newfound workload while leaving just enough time to drive my son to baseball, and my daughter to dance; which of course, were on opposite ends of town.

A couple of months in, I realized I was gaining weight, became more exhausted than normal, had trouble relaxing, and as far as good night's sleep went, forget about it! One particular morning when I woke up, I felt like a truck had hit me. My initial thought was I'm coming down with the flu. I was achy, exhausted, and began to feel as if a breakdown was imminent. I could not get out of bed. When I realized what was actually happening, I almost couldn't believe it. I was so nervous, shaky, and scared, that I could hardly stand up on my own two feet. My family was so worried that they called in the in-laws. The stress had finally won. I was no longer the rock. I couldn't keep up with the demand in my life. If only I would have slowed down to realize what was creeping up on me, I probably could have put a stop to it before it stopped me, literally, in my tracks.

- 1 in 5 Americans experience extreme stress (heart palpitations, shaking, and depression).
- 44% of people say they are more stressed now than they were 5 years ago.
- The American Stress Institute found that 75%–90% of all visits to physicians are due to stress-related complaints.
- Stress increases your risk of heart disease by 40% and risk of stroke by 50%. Yikes!

What is Stress?

Stress is a state of mental or emotional strain, with tension resulting from adverse or very-demanding circumstances. The two different kinds of stress are: short-term or acute stress, and long-term or chronic stress.

- Short-term/Acute Stress: impacts the body for a short amount of time, such as a busy commute home on a busy interstate. In humans and animals alike, this type of stress response can be lifesaving. A deer in the woods hears something, maybe a potential predator, and quickly responds in order to flee a dangerous situation. This is a type of stress which increases your heart rate and breathing while decreasing your digestion. This is also known as the fight-or-flight response, which your body has the ability to quickly recover from.

— Long-term/Chronic Stress: is associated with tremendous amounts negative and lasting health implications. The human body was not designed to be in a constant state of stress. Imagine going through acute stress over and over in a never ending cycle, the body gets exhausted, organs and systems break down easily, and your immune system gets shot. Most people with stress-related health problems suffer from chronic stress.

What Should I Look For?

Stress presents itself differently in men and women. Studies have shown that men can have more anger or aggression when reacting to stress, whereas women have a tendency to want to verbally work out stressful situations by talking.

Physical signs of stress (chronic stress):

- decreased energy
- headaches
- stomach and intestinal upset (which could be nausea, diarrhea, or constipation)
- frequent illnesses
- decreased sexual desire
- high blood pressure, heart problems
- diabetes, skin conditions
- asthma
- arthritis
- clenched jaw
- dry mouth
- shortness of breath or feeling like you can't take a deep breath

Mental signs of stress are:

- depression
- anxiety
- easily agitated/frustrated
- feeling overwhelmed
- difficulty relaxing
- low self-esteem
- loneliness

- avoiding others

Other Conditions to Rule Out:

With the many signs of stress, the recognition and identification of what types are most important. Many different health issues can arise from being under chronic stress and it's easy to overlook, often thinking, "This is just how stressful my life always is, I'm used to it." The body was not designed to handle chronic stress, and for that reason it has a huge negative impact on health. Mental disorders and other issues, like substance abuse, also should be taken into consideration when examining stress levels.

What Puts Me More at Risk?

Having a high-stress job and lifestyle are the two main risk factors for chronic stress. It's important to take a minute and ask yourself what type of stress you have. Be honest with yourself. The only person it is going to matter to is *you*. Sometimes the effects won't show up for a long time, but when that day comes, you will wish you had recognized it earlier.

We all have stress in our day;
the key is to not let it run or ruin your life

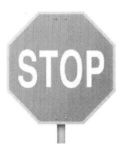

Stop Your Day

If you realize you've had racing thoughts and worry for weeks that has made taking a deep breath more difficult—change your pattern immediately. Make a plan to get out of the stress cycle, even if you have to wait a week to have some time to de-stress.

Diagnostic Tests:

Stress surveys taken monthly or quarterly track your results over time to gauge your stress levels at different points in your life. It's very common to have stress levels peak at certain times of the year. It's important to recognize this stress, and formulate a plan to lower it in other areas of your life.

When I was in graduate school, the stress of studying for midterms, boards, and finals all in a row, would take a toll on my body. I often found, that as soon as I would break for the semester, I would become sick. It's the same as if you are waiting to take a vacation, and when that finally happens, you get sick, which can ruin the time that was scheduled to be stress free in the first place. Becoming sick when there is a break from the normal routine, is an indicator that you suffer from chronic stress.

How Do I Prevent Stress?

The tough thing is that you can't prevent all kinds of stress all the time. Stress is going to happen in your life, it happens to all of us. The stronger your health and immune system are, the easier it is for your body to handle the stress in life, while not causing additional damage to your health along the way.

- Regular exercise (5 days a week for 20 minutes, such as a walk or jog), meditation, and a diet that is non-inflammatory can help to prevent stress. A non-inflammatory diet is one that limits sugar, red meat, dairy, and gluten. You may feel stressed just reading that, but after a couple of weeks, *you will* feel the physical differences. Yoga is also a great tension reliever physically and mentally.

- Meditation not only reduces but also decreases the health dangers associated with stress. It may seem tough for you to meditate at first, keep trying, it takes practice.

- Proper sleep is essential to decrease stress. When you sleep, the body has the opportunity to rest and repair, allowing cells to recover from any strain or pressure you encountered during the day.
- Essential oils, such as lavender, can help decrease stress and tension in your body. Lavender and other oils can be applied to the skin, back, neck, and bottoms of the feet. The use of coconut oil as a medium helps the essential oils soak in.
- Take your vitamins—see list in heart disease. Vitamin D helps with mood and immune system, so take it daily.
-

Bodywork also has advantageous effects on stress. Massages, chiropractic adjustments, and acupuncture can greatly reduce stress levels, especially if performed on a regular basis.

Stop the madness and break the chronic stress cycle. Plan time to break out of your routine of worry, which means doing something out of the ordiQuestions to Ask Yourself:

Have you suffered from stress that you felt you couldn't control?

Have you ever been on medications for stress?

Have you changed anything in your life related to concerns about your stress?

Were you aware women's symptoms were different than men's?

Health Condition No. 5:
Mental Health

I kept waiting for my depression to get better on its own, never thinking it would get worse before it got better.

Since the day I left for college, I've always had a hard time adjusting to new environments. I would eventually get used to the changes, but it would usually take a bit of time. Once I would get settled into a routine, I would get back to feeling like "myself" and doing the things I loved to do. Painting was one of my passions I started in college, which lead to my art major, and was one of the things I could always turn to as an outlet. It would help me calm down after a stressful day, and mostly it made me flat-out happy.

It seemed like every time I had a big change in my life, the period of not feeling like me would last just a little bit longer. Finally, the day came when I lost someone close to me. I can recall days where it would take so much energy just to get out of bed, much less do anything more than what was absolutely necessary to survive. I stopped meeting friends on the weekends, I quit my book club, and most significantly I stopped painting. I came to the realization   that what I was experiencing was depression

This was something I thought I could easily overcome, but didn't think about how tough it would be until my manager pulled me into her office. She stated how I had become completely un-engaged over the last 4–5 months, and my work performance was starting to take a serious nosedive. I went from being the top performer on my team to being dead last. My manager said she wasn't sure what was going on, but whatever it was, I should get some expert help for it. How embarrassing. I thought I could kick this "funk" on my own because I had been able to in the past. I decided against my boss' advice thinking, "Someday I will magically wake up and feel like I am back to normal."

Of course that never happened. I was fired a month later. I don't think I had really done any work in the last six months anyway and was surprised it didn't happen sooner. Most would say this was a blessing in disguise. Now I truly realized how bad my depression had gotten, and that I wasn't going to just "kick it on my own" this time. I needed the expert help that my boss had suggested over a month ago. I was out of a job, all because I waited to get help

- Almost 46 million Americans report a mental illness, yet less than 40% of them get treated.
- Mental Health is linked to stress and affects men and women very differently.
- Men will have more physical symptoms: fatigue, irritability, and sleep problems.
- Women will have more negative emotions, such as guilt, and can experience mental health decline around their menstrual cycle or with winter seasons.
- After giving birth, 10%–16% of postpartum women experience depression.

What is Mental Health?

Mental health is a person's psychological and emotional well-being. The term mental health covers a wide range of conditions, with the most common being depression and anxiety.

- Depression is a medical condition with persistent feelings of sadness and loss of interest.

- Anxiety is a nervous disorder with feelings of worry and nervousness. A person with anxiety can have compulsive behavior and/or panic attacks.

Should I Look For?

Depression can bring feelings of helplessness and hopelessness, along with a loss of interest in daily activities.

- A person with depression can have a change in appetite and/or weight (gain and loss).
- A change in sleep, either a need for excessive sleep or insomnia.
- Mood changes, having anger or irritability, loss of energy, difficulty concentrating, and unexplained aches and pains are physical signs of depression.

Anxiety presents with feelings of panic, fear, uneasiness, shortness of breath, heart palpitations, and episodes that can mimic heart-attack symptoms.

Other Conditions to Rule Out:

It's important to rule out other mental and mood disorders to make sure that when treatment has begun, the correct condition is targeted, allowing you to achieve the fastest result. Depression can be situational depending on the type of event that triggers it. For example, when a loved one dies depression can be accompanied with a period of mourning that eventually fades as time passes, with the hope that the depression will quickly run its course. People do not immediately see the need for help, which only increases the likelihood of the depression becoming chronic.

What Puts Me More at Risk?

- Family history of depression or anxiety
- History of depression and/or anxiety in your past, as well as having a severe chronic illness
- Substance use (alcohol or drugs)
- Environmental circumstances
- Diet and nutrition
- Certain medications can also put you more at risk
- Stress can be a huge factor for depression and anxiety

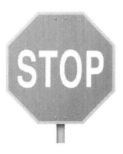

Stop Your Day

Depression can really hit anyone, at any age. If you or anyone you know are showing signs, it's important to take some action. Seek the advice of a health care or counseling professional. Not seeking help can make the mental health issue a lot worse in a short amount of time, making it more difficult to treat. When a diagnosis is made, and treatment is started sooner, improvement is noticed faster.

Diagnostic Tests:

Many screenings and surveys are available for depression and anxiety. Be sure to continue using the same one to track progress through any type of program. Ask your doctor for more information and help.

How Do I Prevent Mental Health Issues?

- Eating a clean diet, one without processed foods, sugars, dairy or gluten.
- Physical activity boosts your endorphins; just 10 minutes of intense movement

(such as H.I.I.T.) can release those fantastic mood-boosting chemicals in your body. Interval training has many health benefits and just 10 minutes a day can boost mental health. A 20-minute walk or yoga are also helpful.

- Regular massage, acupuncture, and chiropractic care are positive ways to help manage and treat depression and anxiety. The hands-on aspect of these therapies assist in many mental health conditions by releasing endorphins during treatment.

- Take your vitamins. Vitamin D is known for boosting mood, and can help with depression.

Questions to Ask Yourself:

Has anyone in your family been diagnosed with a mental health condition?

Have you or are you using medication(s) for mental health issues?

Have you changed anything in your life related to concerns about depression or anxiety?

When was the last time you experienced mental health-related symptoms that you ignored?

Health Condition No. 6: Pain

I thought my pain would get better if I just waited it out.

I woke up one morning with a sore neck, and assumed I slept on it wrong. It's happened before, and it has always gone away. I rubbed it, took a hot shower and got my day started. As I moved around, it seemed to be less severe. We were at the end of a quarter at work, and I knew it was going to be a long couple weeks. On top of this, my mom has just been diagnosed with cancer, and I was trying to carve out time to take her to appointments. Three weeks had gone by before I realized that the top of my neck had become significantly worse, and was accompanied by headaches. I had tried a few quick remedies such as anti-inflammatories and pain cream, but that seemed like a waste of time and money as it didn't even make a dent in my pain.

Two more weeks had gone by, things were slowing down at work—or as much as they could. I remember thinking, "Why does my arm keep falling asleep?" It wasn't until I stopped to actually think about it, that I realized it wasn't "asleep", it was numb all the way down to my fingers. Never before had I experienced a numbness like *this that made using my computer and picking up the phone excruciatingly painful. I knew I needed to go to my doctor, and I had waited too long.*

- Everyone has experienced physical pain at some point in his or her life.
- 31 million Americans suffer from low-back pain at any given time, the most common pain condition in the US.
- People wait years before getting their pain treated, which often causes the treatment to take longer to have the desired effect.

What is Pain?

Many of us have been taught at an early age "No Pain, No Gain". It's become natural throughout our lives to dismiss pain as a necessary evil if we want to get "This Result" or do "That Job", and frankly, we've gotten quite good at hiding it. There are many types of pain that exist in the body, coming from different sources. When most people think of pain, they think of acute trauma—like a slip and fall. Micro-trauma is a small degree of damage that occurs over time and can be very damaging, such as carpel tunnel from excessive computer use. These types of injuries can take a long time to treat and heal due to the length of time it took to develop, as well as the amount of scar tissue now built up in the body.

What Should I Look For?

You should be aware of severe pain in your body, anywhere in your body. It may sound like a silly thing to keep track of—you're thinking "how could I *not* notice when I'm in pain"—but the truth is that many people underestimate how long they have been in pain, which undercuts the severity of the problem. Pain that is rated above a 6 out of 10 on the pain scale that does not improve after 2 days, shouldn't be ignored. Any numbness or tingling anywhere in your body is not normal and should be tracked as well, because it can take a long time to treat. A decrease in your normal range of motion can be a sign to future problems even if you're not having pain from it right away.

Other Conditions to Rule Out:

When your body is in pain, it's trying to tell you there is a problem, but often the actual source of the problem is not exactly where you feel the pain. In fact, 80% of musculoskeletal pain presents itself in an area away from the source of the pain.

This indicates that most of the time where you feel pain in your body isn't the area that needs to be treated. Nerves branch out from your spinal cord, and travel everywhere in your body. If there is pressure on a nerve, the pain can show itself anywhere this nerve travels.

What Puts Me at Risk?

- Growth spurts and pregnancy are risk factors because your body is growing at a fast rate. Your nervous system needs time to adjust to its new body dimensions making you more prone to clumsiness and injuries.
- Stress can cause aches and pains all over the body.
- Bad posture can wear out the joints in your body over time, and cause your muscles to be overworked because the muscles that have to hold the structure in that bad position. The muscles then get fatigued and very sore, which makes you more likely to injure yourself.
- Any diseases or health conditions you may have are risk factors.

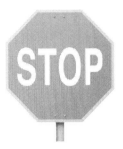

Stop Your Day

Seek attention if you have severe pain, can't move part of your body, can't feel part of your body, the pain is getting worse, or you have other symptoms (loss of bowel/bladder control, chest pain, etc.). If you have had pain that rates a 6 out of 10 or more on the pain scale for more than 1 or 2 days, seek immediate care from a physician.

Now is the time to start treating the pain.

Diagnostic Tests:

Pain index numbers can be helpful to track how much pain you are experiencing over a period of time. If an issue has persisted for a week or so, it can be difficult to remember how severe the pain was five days ago, especially if it has been getting worse. The best thing to do is to ask someone who is close to you. I have frequently seen that people will say they have been in pain for two weeks, and their significant other will say the pain has really been bothering them for a month. Most people are likely to underestimate the problem, especially if it will be a challenge to take care of the pain.

How Do I Prevent Pain?

- Stay healthy, maintain a healthy diet, and exercise. The healthier you are, the better your body will heal from any pain you have and not cause any major damage to your health in the process.
- Eat a diet that is non-inflammatory, and exercise regularly.
- Yoga is great for increasing flexibility and providing a low-impact way to exercise. If yoga doesn't interest you, then a simple walk or swim is a great way to get your body moving with very low impact.
- Posture, posture, posture. Your mom didn't remind you to have good posture just to nag you. Studies have shown that the better your posture is, the healthier you are.
- Regular bodywork, such as massage, chiropractic, and acupuncture are extremely effective in treating and preventing pain in the body. If you haven't tried it yet, get to it! Chiropractic care has been shown to be the most

cost-effective and efficient way to treat low-back pain.

- Essential oils can immediately decrease certain pain in the body. A blend of rosemary, lavender, and peppermint are fantastic for because they decrease sharp pain quickly.

- Take your top 4 supplements daily: Specifically for healing—Vitamin D has also been shown to increase the rate of healthy cell reproduction in higher levels, which translates to your body likely healing faster.

Questions to Ask Yourself:

Have you suffered from pain for more than 48 hours without seeking treatment?

Have you or are you using medications for pain, either over the counter or prescription?

Have you changed anything in your life related to concerns about pain?

Have you noticed a new numbness/tingling sensation anywhere in the body?

Health Condition No. 7:

COPD

I quit smoking ten years ago, so how could I have lung problems now?

I grew up at a time when it seemed like everyone smoked, and we didn't have scary ads telling us what actually happens if you continue to smoke. When I quit, I threw away my pack-a-day habit. A while ago I noticed a cough that seemed slightly different than what I was used to, but having been a smoker for thirty years, it was similar to what I had experienced in the past. I have three very busy grandkids I watch during the week. By Friday I am always exhausted, but it's so worth it. While keeping up with them is becoming harder, I figured it is due to my age.

When my daughter pointed out that my mucus-filled cough had been going on for a while, I realized it had actually been months. In addition to the cough, I was starting to experience tightness in my chest and I always seemed to be short of breath. Again, I thought all of these had to be a cause of aging—and were normal. Just to make sure it wasn't anything serious, I finally decided to see the doctor. I *was taken aback when he told me I had COPD. If only I had gone in sooner, my lungs wouldn't be as damaged.*

- COPD is very common, affecting 24 million Americans each year.
- Today, more women than men die of COPD each year.
- Smoking is the #1 cause of COPD, but 10%–20% of people with COPD have never smoked.
- Over half of the people with COPD are not aware they have it because they ignore the symptoms.
- 70% of COPD sufferers are in the workforce today.

What is COPD?

Chronic Obstructive Pulmonary Disease (COPD) is a group of lung diseases that blocks airflow, making it continually more difficult to breathe. Once the disease has onset it progressively gets worse over time. Emphysema, chronic bronchitis, and non-reversible asthma are all types of COPD.

What Should I Look For?

- Look for coughing that produces large amounts of mucus and wheezing, shortness of breath, or tightening of the chest
- Contracting other illnesses often (like colds and flu)
- Swelling in feet, ankles, legs, and other musculoskeletal pain, combined with the coughing
- Be aware of any treatment for a cough that isn't providing you with a result you think you should be getting, or if the treatment isn't working

We've all seen those pictures of a lung that has become black from smoking next to a healthy pink lung. If only it were that easy to see what's happening within our own bodies, we'd be able to see how much damage we've incurred over time.

Don't guess—because similar to the amount of pain we feel, we usually underestimate how bad things have gotten.

Other Conditions to Rule Out:

Serious conditions such as Congestive Heart Failure (CHF), or other bronchial diseases should be ruled out. Any restricted or decreased breathing warrants an immediate visit to the physician.

What Puts Me More at Risk?

The severity of COPD relates to how much damage you have in your lungs. The damage can result from how long and how often you have smoked. Other risk factors are exposure to second-hand smoke and exposure to chemicals and fumes. Overall health also plays an important role in disease progression, so if you have other chronic diseases or illnesses, like autoimmune diseases, then you are more at risk.

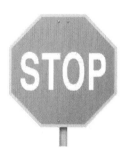

Stop Your Day

If you are having trouble breathing, see your doctor immediately. With COPD the disease continually gets worse. So if you are worried about breathing, the sooner you get help the better. The longer you wait, the harder it is to treat, and the more damage has been done. If you or a loved one works around fine particles or dangerous fumes, ensure the proper use of personal protective equipment at all times.

Attention:
The longer you wait, the harder it is to treat
and the more damage has been done.

Diagnostic Tests:

A breathing test called Spirometry rates how well you are breathing, but most importantly is how you rate your own breathing on a regular basis. Remember, you're not going to last more than about three minutes without air, so as soon as you notice a problem, see a physician.

How Do I Prevent COPD?

- Stop smoking. Don't start smoking or be around smoke.
- Stay away from chemicals, dust, and fumes as much as possible or ensure proper use of personal protective equipment.
- Stay healthy, eat well and exercise. The healthier you are, the better your body can handle illnesses.
- Eat a diet that is non-inflammatory, limiting sugar, red meat, dairy and

gluten. Make sure you are getting 5 vegetable servings a day.

- Yoga is great for increasing flexibility and providing a low-impact way to exercise. A brisk walk or a swim are other great ways to get your body moving with very low impact.

- Massage and chiropractic are very effective at getting the ribcage moving so breathing can be easier.

- Good posture makes breathing easier. Give it a try, slump down in your chair and take a deep breath. It's pretty tough. Now sit up really straight and breathe deep into your lungs. You will notice a huge difference immediately. So keep your posture strong!

- Take your top 4 vitamins every day: Vitamin D also helps to boost the immune system.

Questions to Ask Yourself:

Does anyone in your family have COPD?

Have you had a mucus-producing cough for more than 3 weeks?

Do you or have your ever smoked?

Have you been exposed to second-hand smoke or chemical fumes?

When was your last physical?

Stop Your Day

Health Condition No. 8: Autoimmune Disease

I thought I was going crazy with all the health problems I had—and no one could find a solution.

I went from being a super active 20-year-old, to a 25-year-old who could barely hold a part-time job. A couple months after I completed my first triathlon, it all started. I was constantly tired and fatigued, to the point that simply walking up the stairs became a chore. The first doctor told me it was normal, calling it something like "post-college student fatigue."

This can't be a real thing, can it? I was told college students are so deprived of sleep that when they graduate, their body goes into catch-up mode. Along with the fatigue, I started getting some dry patches on my skin, an onset of digestive issues, and a constant feeling of being cold. It could be 90 degrees in the middle of summer, and I would be wrapped up in a blanket. I knew something was not right.

The second doctor ran a bunch of tests, which all came back as inconclusive. I cut out processed foods and attempted to exercise even when I felt like it was going to put me in bed for the rest of the day. These things helped from time to time, but overall there was *never a drastic change in how I felt. It was kind of like how you feel the day before you get the full- blown flu—Terrible. After five different doctors in as many years, one finally gave me the correct diagnosis of autoimmune disease.*

- More than 50 million Americans have autoimmune disease, and more than 75% of them are women.
- Autoimmune disease is the underlying cause of more than 100 serious and chronic illnesses.

What is Autoimmune Disease?

Autoimmune diseases arise from abnormal immune responses to substances and tissues that are normally present in the body. This imperfection in the immune system occurs in different areas of the body. Your body mounts a defense against something that your body thinks is dangerous—but is actually normal tissue. So essentially, your body is fighting against itself.

What Should I Look For?

Diagnosis can be difficult because the symptoms can vary greatly from person to person, and can affect multiple body systems in different ways. Autoimmune disease is the most poorly understood and recognized category of illness for people. A lot of women who are diagnosed are younger, in their childbearing years, and traditionally thought of as being very healthy.

Things to look for are:

- skin problems
- joint pain or joint problems
- fatigue
- intestinal issues (diarrhea or constipation)
- hair loss
- thyroid problems
- brain fog
- kidney or brain problems
- feeling ill or sick for longer than 3-4 weeks.

Stress can make these symptoms worse at specific times, making the diagnosis even more difficult for physicians.

Other Conditions to Rule Out:

Being diagnosed with an autoimmune disease can take a long time because the symptoms can present so differently in so many different tissues, and can occur for years. On the average, *it takes about 4.6 years and 5 different doctors* for a person to be accurately diagnosed with an autoimmune disease.

It's important to rule out different types of autoimmune diseases to be sure that you are targeting the correct condition. Other illnesses to rule out could be stress, mental health diseases, heart disease, etc.

What Puts Me More at Risk?

The cause of autoimmune diseases is not really known, making the risk factors is hard to identify. Autoimmune diseases tend to run in families. If the health history of your family's past is not well known, track your condition so it is easy to discuss with a physician. Think about it this way, when looking back in time, people didn't go to the doctor unless their arm was falling off or there was a life threatening condition, so your family history may not be complete.

Environmental factors play a part in autoimmune disease, so limit or eliminate your exposure to dangerous chemicals.

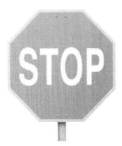

Stop Your Day

Often the patient has to be persistent in getting the help they need. Autoimmune disease symptoms can be all over the board, making it tough to identify the specific condition. Don't get discouraged. *You know* if something is not right with your health, so see a doctor and be persistent to get the answers you need.

Make sure to mention to your physician how a change in your lifestyle affects your autoimmune condition. For example, if you start a non-inflammatory diet and see a great improvement in symptoms, tell your doctor.

Diagnostic Tests:

- Getting your blood tested is a great way to track your health.

- Thyroid blood levels should be tested every 3 months (it takes 3 months for the hormone levels to shift in the body). Keep track of them until there is normal hormone levels are present for 6 straight months.

- Iron levels in your blood can show if you are anemic and if your body is absorbing the nutrients from your food.
- Getting a white and red blood cell count will also let you know if your body is healthy.

How Do I Prevent Autoimmune Disease?

It can be difficult to pinpoint a specific way to prevent autoimmune disease, as a cause hasn't been identified. The healthier you are, and the stronger your immune system is, the fewer symptoms you will experience from any illness. The best ways to build an ironclad immune system are good nutrition, healthy diet, exercise, massage, chiropractic care, and taking supplements. A food elimination diet can be helpful in identifying foods that may aggravate symptoms.

Taking daily vitamins strengthens your immune system. Vitamin D has been shown to boost the immune system, so get your levels checked to make sure you have enough in your system.

Questions to Ask Yourself:

Has anyone in your family been diagnosed with an autoimmune illness?

Have you been to multiple doctors for symptoms that don't seem to be consistent?

Have you used medication for symptoms without a noticeable change?

Have you experienced symptoms that you have ignored?

Stop Your Day

Health Condition No. 9:
Bone Health

I was certain that my bones were too healthy and strong to break.

I left work late on a Friday, and I remember rushing home to get prepared for having a couple of friends over for dinner. It often seems like when you are strapped for time, a million things will get in your way to slow you down. I had forgotten an important ingredient at the grocery store, my car was running low on gas, the dog had an accident on the floor, etc. You know how it goes. I was in the middle of putting together appetizers, setting the table, and greeting my guests when I did something that changed my life forever.

My husband had left a package he received that day in front of the door to the garage, I reached down to pick it up, not realizing how heavy it was, and heard a crunch in my back. It was excruciating. I screamed and fell to the floor in agony. When I got to the ER, they took an X-ray and found a fracture in my spine. I couldn't believe it. I was in my early 50s and otherwise healthy; it didn't make sense to me. When my doctor told me I had osteoporosis, I was at a loss for words.

All I wanted to know was how and why did I get it, and what could have been done to prevent it?

- 54 million Americans live with or are at risk for, osteoporosis and low-bone mass.
- Another 54.2 million Americans have osteoarthritis.
- 60% of all arthritis is found in women.
- 1 out of every 2 women and 1 out of every 4 men over the age of 50 will break a bone due to osteoporosis.

What is Osteoporosis and Osteoarthritis?

Bones are living and growing tissues. It's hard to think of them that way because you can't "see" them growing like you can see your skin grow together when you have a cut. It takes about 6–8 weeks for a bone fracture to heal, with your overall health playing a huge role in how fast that occurs.

Osteoporosis: Weakness and decreased density in bone tissue due to hormone changes and calcium or vitamin D deficiencies.

Osteoarthritis: Degeneration of the cartilage and the bone in a joint that can occur anywhere in the body, but is common in the spine, hips, knees, fingers, and toes. Arthritis can continually get worse if left untreated.

What Should I Look For?

Osteoporosis: back pain, loss of height, stooped posture, or bone fracture. Most people who are at risk of having osteoporosis learn about it after they fall and break their hip.

Osteoarthritis: Pain, stiffness and swelling in a joint after sitting or getting out of bed. Arthritis can be caused by trauma, injury, or overuse of a joint that doesn't get treated.

Other Conditions to Rule Out:

For both osteoporosis and osteoarthritis, rule out other bone diseases, joint diseases, or inflammatory diseases like autoimmune disease.

What Puts Me More at Risk?

- Family history of osteoporosis or osteoarthritis can be a risk factor
- Poor nutrition and lack of exercise
- Certain medications can cause your bones to become weaker and more brittle

- Being overweight is very hard on your joints and bones, and can lead to bone disease
- Smoking and drinking diet soda can leech the calcium and important nutrients out of healthy bone tissues

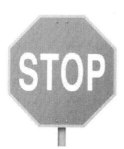

Stop Your Day

Know your bone density numbers and how strong your bones are. If you haven't done weight-bearing activity at least 2–3 times this week, now is the time to start.

Diagnostic Tests:

Bone density score indicates the strength and health of your bones.

- Bone density is measured by a T-score: +1 to -1 is normal. -1 to -2.5 is low, and below -2.5 is considered osteoporotic (osteoporosis of the bone).

- X-rays of a painful area can show if there is arthritis in that specific joint, and blood tests can tell you if arthritis factors are present.

How Do I Prevent Osteoporosis and Osteoarthritis?

- Diet, exercise, and your weight are the biggest factors in preventing bone disease. Get a healthy diet of protein (such as chicken, turkey, and fish) and lots of leafy green vegetables. Calcium is essential, and vegetables like broccoli have high levels of calcium.
- To build bone strength it's important to do some weight-bearing activity. This can be weight lifting in a gym or body-weight exercises like yoga and Pilates.
- Being overweight is the hardest thing for your joints. Getting on a weight reduction program will eventually help to take the pressure off your joints and give them a break that they wouldn't otherwise get.
- Vitamins can ensure your body has the nutrient it needs. The top 4 supplements to take daily are: 1. Multivitamin 2. Fish Oil 3. Probiotic and 4. Vitamin D, which is

necessary for the body to absorb calcium from food or other supplements. (See details in Heart Disease section)

Questions to Ask Yourself:

Has anyone in your family been diagnosed with osteoporosis or osteoarthritis?

Has your doctor commented about your bone health?

Have you ever had an x-ray that showed osteoarthritis in a joint?

When was your last physical?

Have you ever had a bone- density scan?

Stop Your Day

Health Condition No. 10: Addiction

I had heard stories of it happening, but never thought it could happen to me.

I had always been a straight-A student, and by my early twenties had turned into a very successful businesswoman. I followed all the rules, never got into trouble, and my parents thought of me as the golden child. I wouldn't even speed—it just wasn't who I was.

The day my life was changed forever started out like any other day. I was driving to work when out of nowhere I was on the side of the highway, in a smashed up car. I really have no idea what happened. After a trip to the hospital with a broken collarbone, I was sent home to heal with a prescription for painkillers to help keep me comfortable.

Being a healthy young woman helped me heal much faster than what the doctors expected. A month or so after the accident I was back to working full time, and felt like I was on the fast track to being myself again. The doctors had told me to take the painkillers as needed to keep the pain at bay, or until the prescription ran out.

However, after the prescription ran out, I found myself aching for more. A short month on those pills—and I was hooked.

- 1 out of every 8 Americans is addicted to something.
- There is no way to know for certain who will become an addict, and addiction can happen in a very short period of time, even from first-time use.
- Addiction affects 23.2 million Americans, and only 10% receive the treatment they need.

What is Addiction?

Substance Addiction is the compulsive need for and use of any habit-forming substance. With use, a tolerance is built up for the substance, and upon withdrawal, specific physiological symptoms appear.

Behavior Addiction is having a compulsive engagement in an activity despite any negative impacts that behavior has on the person's physical, emotional or financial well-being. Some behavior addictions are gambling, shopping, sex and video games.

What Should I Look For?

If you are addicted, you cannot stop taking the substance or quit the behavior, and if you do stop, withdrawal symptoms begin. Withdrawal symptoms are physical- and mood-related symptoms such as:

- small pupils
- frequent nosebleeds
- change in appetite
- change in sleep patterns
- deterioration in physical appearance
- change and/or increase in body odor
- shakes or tremors.

Other Conditions to Rule Out:

Many substances and behaviors are addictive: alcohol, tobacco, drugs, gambling, shopping, sex, food, video games, Internet, or work. It's important to differentiate between taking a substance for a limited period of time for a purpose (like pain medication following removal of your wisdom teeth) and not being able to stop taking the pain medication even though your mouth has healed.

What Puts Me More at Risk?

- Biological factors include inherited traits that may make you more at risk.
- Environmental risks include any social groups you belong to, and the peers with whom you spend time.
- Development factors include your personal growth and emotional intelligence.

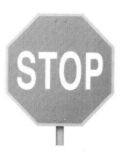

Stop Your Day

Often it's the person with the addiction who can't see that they are addicted. They would need a friend or family member to tell them that the substance has taken over their life, and they need help.

Diagnostic Tests:

Diagnosis requires an evaluation and/or assessment by a licensed professional. There is a specific process to be diagnosed with addiction, and it is vital that this process is thoroughly completed.

How Do I Prevent Becoming Addicted?

- Self-care. The healthier you are, the less likely you will need medications.
- Create a great support system around you, and include a healthy group of people you can count on. Your support group can and should consist of professionals you can trust.
- Continue learning and growing as a person. Volunteering is a great way to expand your personal growth.
- Educate yourself and your friends/family on the signs and damaging effects of addiction.
- Start a lifestyle that is low in stress.
- Seek counseling.
- Maintain friendships with people who are not addicted to substances.
- Be sure to take the top 4 supplements daily as described in Heart Disease section.

Questions to Ask Yourself:

Does anyone in your family have a history of addiction?

Have your friends or family ever commented or been concerned about you being addicted to a substance—or a behavior?

Have you changed anything in your life to continue using a substance?

Start Your Life

Don't wait for your health to stop your day, get to your doctor at the first signs of a condition and make prevention a top priority.

I cannot stress enough the importance of a healthy diet and exercise. The two are an integral part in maintaining health and disease prevention. You cannot expect peak performance from your body if you tolerate inferior fuel.

This book should serve as a guide for women who live busy lives and want be their healthiest. Please connect and share with other important people in your life and be aware of the top health concerns and how to prevent them in your future. Knowing and paying attention to the red flags from the body can mean the difference between life and death.

It's essential to make a very specific distinction in the information women are given that is different from that given to men. Women's health has been left out of the conversation for far too long—and it's time for a change. This book is just the start. When women know what to look for, and when it's absolutely essential to stop their day, more women will be empowered to take control of their health, and ultimately their lives. Join the movement of empowered healthy women, recruit others around you, and start your healthy life.

References:

Stop Your Day – Research

ADDICTION

http://www.webmd.com/mental-health/addiction/features/prescription-drug-abuse-who-gets-addicted-and-why

http://health.clevelandclinic.org/2012/08/6-myths-about-painkillers/

https://ncadd.org/learn-about-drugs/signs-and-symptoms

http://www.medicalnewstoday.com/info/addiction/signs-of-addiction.php

http://www.mayoclinic.org/diseases-conditions/drug-addiction/basics/tests-diagnosis/con-20020970

http://www.drugabuse.gov/publications/drugfacts/understanding-drug-abuse-addiction

http://www.nlm.nih.gov/medlineplus/magazine/issues/spring07/articles/spring07pg14-17.html

http://www.webpsychologist.net/10-most-common-**addictions/**

BONE HEALTH

http://nof.org/

http://www.cdc.gov/arthritis/basics/faqs.htm

AUTOIMMUNE

http://www.aarda.org/autoimmune-information/autoimmune-disease-in-women/

http://www.nlm.nih.gov/medlineplus/autoimmunediseases.html#cat5

http://www.healthline.com/health/autoimmune-disorders

COPD

http://www.nhlbi.nih.gov/health/health-topics/topics/copd

http://www.copdfoundation.org/

http://www.nhlbi.nih.gov/health/health-topics/topics/copd/signs

http://www.lung.org/lung-disease/copd/about-copd/preventing-copd.html

http://www.everydayhealth.com/health-report/chronic-obstructive-pulmonary-disease/benefits-of-early-copd-diagnosis-val-ashbury.aspx

PAIN

http://www.cdc.gov/nchs/fastats/leading-causes-of-death.htm

HEART DISEASE

http://www.nhlbi.nih.gov/health/health-topics/topics/hdw

http://www.mayoclinic.org/diseases-conditions/heart-disease/basics/definition/con-20034056

http://www.nhlbi.nih.gov/health/health-topics/topics/hdw/signs

http://www.mayoclinic.org/diseases-conditions/heart-disease/in-depth/heart-disease/art-20049357

http://www.cdc.gov/women/heart/

https://www.goredforwomen.org/about-heart-disease/facts_about_heart_disease_in_women-sub-category/causes-prevention/

CANCER: LUNG

http://www.lung.org/lung-disease/lung-cancer/resources/facts-figures/lung-cancer-fact-sheet.html

http://www.webmd.com/cancer/features/15-cancer-symptoms-women-ignore

http://lungcancer.about.com/od/whatislungcancer/a/lungcancerwomen.htm

http://health.usnews.com/health-news/health-wellness/articles/2013/11/15/a-medical-mystery-why-is-lung-cancer-rising-among-nonsmoking-women

http://www.cancer.gov/cancertopics/types/lung

DIABETES

http://www.merriam-webster.com/dictionary/diabetes

http://www.diabetes.org/diabetes-basics/symptoms/

http://www.cdc.gov/diabetes/pubs/statsreport14/national-diabetes-report-web.pdf

http://www.cdc.gov/diabetes/pubs/pdf/womenHighRiskDiabetes.pdf

STRESS

http://www.webmd.boots.com/stress-management/physical-stress-symptoms

http://www.helpguide.org/articles/depression/depression-signs-and-symptoms.htm

http://www.webmd.com/anxiety-panic/guide/mental-health-anxiety-disorders

http://usatoday30.usatoday.com/news/health/medical/
health/medical/mentalhealth/story/2012-01-19/Many-
with-mental-illness-go-without-treatment-survey-
says/52653166/1

http://www.stress.org/stress-is-killing-you/

MENTAL HEALTH

http://www.helpguide.org/articles/depression/depressi
on-signs-and-symptoms.htm

http://www.nimh.nih.gov/health/topics/depression/ind
ex.shtml

http://www.webmd.com/anxiety-panic/guide/mental-
health-anxiety-disorders

http://www.adaa.org/

http://www.mentalhealth.gov/

Made in the USA
San Bernardino, CA
24 April 2019